# TRUE KETO
# SMOOTHIES & SHAKES

## 40 Recipes

### Low Carb   High Fat

**Varied Levels of Protein to Cater for All Protein Intake Requirements**

**Formulated By A Dietician Specifically For The Ketogenic Diet**

by Skye Howard RD LD

©Authored by Skye Howard RD LD
Published December 2014 - SCG Publishing
This Edition March 2016

ISBN-13: 978-1530150212
ISBN-10: 1530150213

## DISCLAIMER

# CONTENTS

# Introduction

Are you looking for a quick, Ketogenic-friendly snack or meal to go? You are in for a treat with this Ketogenic Smoothie Recipe Book, which includes 40 Ketogenic smoothies that provide adequate fat and low carbohydrate to help you achieve your personalized health and wellness goals.

With 11 recipes providing under 4g carbs, 9 providing 5-7g carbs, and 14 providing 8-10g carbs, (note all carbs are net) you will never go hungry. Developed by a registered and licensed dietician, they are true to the Ketogenic diet, with accurate nutritional analysis.

There is also a range of protein grams in these recipes, from low to moderate, depending on what your needs are. Athletes and those who exercise will require more protein than those who are sedentary.

The 40 recipes include a variety of flavors and textures to satisfy your palate, including superfoods such as kale, berries, spinach, cocoa, coconut, beets and chia, and with a large variety of other ingredients ranging from almond and coconut milk, MCT oil, coffee, pumpkin and peppermint, to name a few.

Features of the Dietician-Approved Ketogenic Cookbook include:

- 40 dietician approved flavorful and colorful smoothie recipes
- Nutrient analysis for every recipe, including total calories, fat, net carbohydrates and protein

- Recipes categorised into:
  - Under 5g carbs
  - 5g-7g carbs
  - 8g-10g carbs
  - 11-15g carbs
- Includes super foods such as spinach, kale, chia seeds, blueberries and avocado
- Includes Stevia, a natural sweetener derived from the leaves of the plant species Stevia rebaudiana.
- Includes MCT Oil, known as Medium-Chain Triglycerides, which is beneficial for those on the Ketogenic diet because it is:
  - Easily absorbed and aids fat digestion
  - Promotes ketosis
  - Is a quick fuel to organs and muscles

To receive personalized nutritional advice on the proper ratio of fat, carbohydrates and protein, please consult with your local Registered Dietician. For medical advice, please consult your healthcare physician.

# EXPLANATION OF CARBOHYDRATE ANALYSIS

Analysing nutrient values of recipes is somewhat complex. The precise way is to first subtract all of the insoluble fiber from the total carbs and total fiber. If there are more than 5 grams of total fiber remaining, you can also subtract half of the remaining fiber from total carbs. Next it is necessary to assess the sugar alcohols. If there are more than 5 grams, subtract half that amount from the total carbohydrates. If erythritol is the only sugar alcohol listed, you may not subtract any sugar alcohols.

The nutritional analyses of the recipes in this book have been prepared by a registered and licenced dietician who is currently studying for her Masters in Nutrition. She prepared the recipes herself and you can rest assured her recipe analyses are accurate and precise.

# EXPLANATION OF PROTEIN REQUIREMENTS ON THE KETOGENIC DIET

Based on numerous studies, a good range for daily protein intake is 1.5 - 2.0 grams per kilogram of bodyweight, or 0.7 - 0.9 grams per pound.

For macronutrient ranges, typically 5-10% of calories come from carbs, 15-30% from protein and 65-75% from fat. The exact amount of fat and protein is a matter of individual body responses and activity levels. However, most people on ketogenic diets don't consume of 5% of calories from carbohydrates, and protein intake is moderate.

Note: For personalised intake, speak with a Registered Dietician on your specific protein needs per day and per meal. As a guide and quick analysis, there are many free online Keto calculators, such as the KetoDiet Buddy.

# Why is protein so important for weight loss?

There are a number of reasons for maintaining the correct protein levels in your Ketogenic Diet:

1. Evidence proves that protein is most sating for hunger. Being on the Keto diet it is crucial to avoid hunger and one of the easiest ways to avoid carbohydrate craving is to include the correct amount of protein as well as fat in your diet.

2. Evidence also proves that you will burn more calories keeping your diet rich in protein as it increases energy expenditure.

3. Protein is the most important macronutrient for building and preserving muscle tissue, especially for those physically active. And the more muscles you have, the more calories you will burn, even when resting.

# How much protein do you need?

Getting a minimum intake of protein is optimal to prevent muscle wasting at 0.8 g/kg body weight. Studies have shown that males maintained their lean muscle mass at 1.4 g /kg body weight and females at 1.2 g/kg. This means that a 150 lb./68kg female needs 82 g grams of protein per day and a 200 lb./90kg male needs on average about 130 grams of protein per day. Therefore, a larger individual may need more protein at a meal than someone else.

The recipes in this book have been written to provide varying ranges of protein along with low carbohydrates, for the differing needs of individuals, such as athletes who will require more grams of protein over an adult who gets less activity. Protein needs vary and need to be personalised, based on height, weight, gender, age, and activity. Remember you can check online calculators for your personalized protein intake requirements, and base your meal plans on this.

# Can too much protein take you out of Ketosis?

There is no known amount of protein that is shown to interfere with ketosis as everyone responds to protein intake differently, so this is highly personalised. When you eat more protein than your body needs or "excessive intake", some of the amino acids in the protein will be turned into glucose via a process called gluconeogenesis. The glucogenic amino acid is known as alanine. However, moderate protein, very low-carb and high fat will likely prevent this.

The smoothie and shakes recipes in this book are not meant to serve as excessive protein choices. There are a few recipes that are quite high in protein, however, everyone needs different protein amounts and some people would be looking for higher protein intake.

# XANTHAM GUM

Xanthan gum is a universally well-known thickener that has become increasingly popular. It is a corn-based thickener and binder and is used by many reputable ketogenic recipe websites using whole foods, which includes this recipe book. It is high in soluble fiber and stable which makes it great for smoothies, and results in lower net carbs. You could replace the xantham gum with a thickener of your own choice, but you then need to recalculate the nutritional analysis.

# STEVIA

Stevia is a natural sweetener derived from the leaves of the plant species Stevia rebaudiana. It comes in liquid, powder or tablet form. It is possible to grow stevia in your garden, then simply grind finely when the plant is mature.

# MTC OIL

MCT Oil, known as Medium-Chain Triglycerides is beneficial by those on the Ketogenic diet as it is:

- Easily absorbed and aids with fat digestion
- Promotes ketosis
- Is a quick fuel to organs and muscles

If you wish to add MCT oil to your diet, use 1 tbsp. to start of MCT and gradually increase to 2 tbsp., if desired, after 1-2 weeks. This will allow optimal digestion from stomach.

For extra fat in any of the recipes, add 1 tbsp. (15ml) MCT Oil. 1 tbsp. contains 100 calories, provides 100 calories from fat, with a total fat content of 14g (all saturated).

Skye Howard

# SMOOTHIES & SHAKES
# UNDER 5G CARBS

## CREAMY CHOCOLATE MILKSHAKE                  11
Calories: 292
Fat: 25 g
Carbohydrates: 4 g
Protein: 15 g


## FAT BURNING ESPRESSO SMOOTHIE              12
Calories: 270.5
Fat: 16 g
Carbohydrates: 2 g
Protein: 30 g


## BLUEBERRY BLISS                            13
Calories: 302
Fat: 25 g
Carbohydrates: 4 g
Protein: 15 g


## CINNAMON ROLL SMOOTHIE                     14
Calories: 145
Fat: 3.25 g
Carbohydrates: 1.6 g
Protein: 0.6 g


## BLUEBERRY AVOCADO SMOOTHIE                 15
Calories: 377
Fat: 22.5 g
Carbohydrates: 4 g
Protein: 32 g

BLACKBERRY CHOCOLATE SHAKE 16
Calories: 338
Fat: 34 g
Carbohydrates: 4 g
Protein: 1 g

PUMPKIN PIE BUTTERED COFFEE 17
Calories: 120
Fat: 12 g
Carbohydrates: 2 g
Protein: 1 g

CUCUMBER SPINACH SMOOTHIE 18
Calories: 335
Fat: 33 g
Carbohydrates: 4 g
Protein: 3 g

ORANGE CREAMSICLE 19
Calories: 290
Fat: 25 g
Carbohydrates: 4 g
Protein: 15 g

CAYENNE CHOCOLATE SHAKE 20
Calories: 258
Fat: 26 g
Carbohydrates: 3 g
Protein: 3 g

SHAMROCK SHAKE 21
Calories: 195
Fat: 19.5 g
Carbohydrates: 4.5 g
Protein: 2 g

# CREAMY CHOCOLATE MILKSHAKE

A high fat, extremely low carb, low to moderate protein shake.

Makes: 2 servings
Serving size: 8 oz.

**Nutritional Information** (Per serving):

Calories: 292
Fat: 25 g
Carbohydrates: 4 g
Protein: 15 g

**All you need:**

16 oz. unsweetened almond milk, vanilla
1 packet stevia
4 oz. heavy cream
1 scoop Whey Isolate Chocolate protein powder
½ cup crushed ice

**All you do:**

Add all ingredients into blender and blend until smooth.

# FAT BURNING ESPRESSO SMOOTHIE

An extremely low carb (2g), high fat, higher protein smoothie, for those with higher protein requirements.

Makes: 1 serving
Serving size: 1 cup

**Nutritional Information** (Per serving):

Calories: 270.5
Fat: 16 g
Carbohydrates: 2 g
Protein: 30 g

**All you need:**

1 scoop Isopure Zero Carb protein powder
1 espresso shot
¼ c Greek yogurt, full fat
Liquid stevia, to sweeten
Pinch of cinnamon
5 ice cubes

**All you do:**

Add all ingredients into blender and blend until smooth.

# BLUEBERRY BLISS

A high fat, low carb, moderate protein smoothie, depending on your protein requirements.

Makes: 2 servings
Serving size: 10 oz.

**Nutritional Information** (Per serving):

Calories: 302
Fat: 25 g
Carbohydrates: 4 g
Protein: 15 g

**All you need:**

16 oz. unsweetened almond milk, vanilla
1 packet stevia
4 oz. heavy cream
1 scoop Whey Isolate Vanilla protein powder
¼ cup frozen blueberries, unsweetened

**All you do:**

Add all ingredients into blender and blend until smooth.

# CINNAMON ROLL SMOOTHIE

An all-round extremely low carb (1.6g), low fat and low protein smoothie, to add variety to your daily diet. To increase the fat in this recipe add 1 tbsp. MCT Oil. This will add 100 calories and 14g fat (0 carbs, 0 proteins).

Makes: 1 serving
Serving size: 4 oz.

**Nutritional Information** (Per serving):

Calories: 145
Fat: 3.25 g
Carbohydrates: 1.6 g
Protein: 0.6 g

**All you need:**

1 cup unsweetened almond milk
2 tbsp. vanilla protein powder
½ tsp cinnamon
¼ tsp vanilla extract
1 packet stevia
1 tbsp. chia seeds
1 cup ice cubes

**All you do:**

Add all ingredients into blender and blend until smooth.

# BLUEBERRY AVOCADO SMOOTHIE

An extremely low carb (4g), high fat, higher protein smoothie, for those with higher protein requirements.

Makes: 2 servings
Serving size: 6 oz.

**Nutritional Information** (Per serving):

Calories: 377
Fat: 22.5 g
Carbohydrates: 4 g
Protein: 32 g

**All you need:**

1 cup unsweetened almond milk, vanilla
1 tbsp. heavy cream
½ avocado, peeled, pitted, sliced
1 scoop Isopure Coconut Zero Carb protein powder
¼ cup frozen blueberries, unsweetened
Liquid stevia, to sweeten

**All you do:**

Add all ingredients into blender and blend until smooth.

# BLACKBERRY CHOCOLATE SHAKE

An extremely low carb (4g), high fat, and extremely low protein (1g) shake. Ensure you make up your daily meal protein intake through other dietary sources.

Makes: 2 servings
Serving size: 5 oz.

**Nutritional Information** (Per serving):

Calories: 338
Fat: 34 g
Carbohydrates: 4 g
Protein: 1 g

**All you need:**

1 cup unsweetened coconut milk
¼ cup fresh blackberries
2 tbsp. cacao powder
Liquid stevia, to sweeten
6 ice cubes
¼ tsp xanthan gum
1-2 tbsp. MCT oil

Use 1 tbsp. of MCT to start and gradually increase to 2 tbsp., if desired, after 1-2 weeks. This will allow optimal digestion from stomach.

**All you do:**

Add all ingredients into blender and blend until smooth.

# PUMPKIN PIE BUTTERED COFFEE

An all-round extremely low carb (2g), lower fat and extremely low protein (1g) smoothie, to add variety to your daily diet. Ensure you make up your daily protein intake through other dietary sources. To increase the fat in this recipe add 1 tbsp. MCT Oil. This will add 100 calories and 14g fat (0 carbs, 0 proteins).

Makes: 1 serving
Serving size: 12 oz.

**Nutritional Information** (Per serving):

Calories: 120
Fat: 12 g
Carbohydrates: 2 g
Protein: 1 g

**All you need:**

12 oz. hot coffee
2 tbsp. canned pumpkin
1 tbsp. regular butter, unsalted
¼ tsp pumpkin pie spice
Liquid stevia, to sweeten

**All you do:**

Add all ingredients into blender and blend until frothy.

# CUCUMBER SPINACH SMOOTHIE

A high fat, low carb (4g) and low protein (3g) smoothie. Ensure to you make up your daily protein intake through other dietary sources.

Makes: 1 serving
Serving size: 10 oz.

**Nutritional Information** (Per serving):

Calories: 335
Fat: 33 g
Carbohydrates: 4 g
Protein: 3 g

**All you need:**

2 large handfuls spinach
½ cucumber, peeled and cubed
6 ice cubes
1 cup coconut milk
Liquid stevia, to sweeten
¼ tsp xanthan gum
1-2 tbsp. MCT oil

**All you do:**

Add all ingredients into blender and blend until spinach is no longer chunky.

# ORANGE CREAMSICLE

A high fat, low carb (4g) and moderate protein shake.

Makes: 2 servings
Serving size: 10 oz.

**Nutritional Information** (Per serving):

Calories: 290
Fat: 25 g
Carbohydrates: 4 g
Protein: 15 g

**All you need:**

16 oz. unsweetened almond milk, vanilla
1 packet stevia
4 oz. heavy cream
1 scoop Whey Isolate Tropical Dreamsicle protein powder
½ cup crushed ice

**All you do:**

Add all ingredients into blender and blend until smooth.

# CAYENNE CHOCOLATE SHAKE

A high fat, low carb (3g), and low protein shake. Ensure to make up your daily protein requirements through other dietary sources.

Makes: 2 servings
Serving size: 5 oz.

**Nutritional Information** (Per serving):
Calories: 258
Fat: 26 g
Carbohydrates: 3 g
Protein: 3 g

**All you need:**

¼ cup coconut cream
2 tbsp. unrefined coconut oil
1 tbsp. whole chia seeds, spectrum
2 tbsp. cacao
Dash of vanilla extract
Pinch of ground cinnamon
½ pinch cayenne powder
½ - 1 cup water
Ice cubes, if desired

**All you do:**

Add all ingredients into blender and blend until smooth.

# SHAMROCK SHAKE

A high fat, low carb, low protein shake. Ensure to make up your daily protein requirements through other dietary sources.

Makes: 4 servings
Serving size: 1 cup

**Nutritional Information** (Per serving):

Calories: 195
Fat: 19.5 g
Carbohydrates: 4.5 g
Protein: 2 g

**All you need:**

1 cup coconut milk, unsweetened
1 avocado, peeled, pitted, sliced
Liquid stevia, to sweeten
1 cup ice
1 tbsp. pure vanilla extract
1 tsp pure peppermint extract

**All you do:**

Add all ingredients into blender and blend until smooth.

Skye Howard

# SMOOTHIES & SHAKES
# 5G - 7G CARBS

CHAI COCONUT SHAKE                          25
Calories: 233
Fat: 20 g
Carbohydrates: 5 g
Protein: 4 g


AVOCADO ALMOND SMOOTHIE                      26
Calories: 252
Fat: 18 g
Carbohydrates: 5 g
Protein: 17 g


STRAWBERRY ALMOND DELIGHT                    27
Calories: 304
Fat: 25 g
Carbohydrates: 7 g
Protein: 15 g


CREAMY BLACKBERRY                            28
Calories: 237.5
Fat: 22 g
Carbohydrates: 6 g
Protein: 2.3 g10


PEANUT BUTTER MILKSHAKE                       29
Calories: 253
Fat: 23.8 g
Carbohydrates: 7 g
Protein: 5.5 g10

## RASPBERRY SMOOTHIE                     30
Calories: 285
Fat: 22 g
Carbohydrates: 7 g
Protein: 14.5 g


## LEPRECHAUN SHAKE                       31
Calories: 217
Fat: 13 g
Carbohydrates: 7.5 g
Protein: 13 g


## BREAKFAST EGG SMOOTHIE                 32
Calories: 266
Fat: 17 g
Carbohydrates: 6.3 g
Protein: 22.6 g


## PEANUT BUTTER CARAMEL SHAKE           33
Calories: 366
Fat: 35 g
Carbohydrates: 6 g
Protein: 7 g

# CHAI COCONUT SHAKE

A high fat, low carb, low protein shake. Ensure to make up your daily protein requirements through other dietary sources.

Makes: 2 servings
Serving size: 5 oz.

**Nutritional Information** (Per serving):

Calories: 233
Fat: 20 g
Carbohydrates: 5 g
Protein: 4 g

**All you need:**

1 cup unsweetened coconut milk
1 tbsp. pure vanilla extract
2 tbsp. almond butter
¼ cup unsweetened shredded coconut
1 tsp ground ginger
1 tsp ground cinnamon
Pinch of allspice
1 tbsp. ground flaxseed
5 ice cubes

**All you do:**

Add all ingredients into blender and blend until smooth.

# AVOCADO ALMOND SMOOTHIE

A high fat, low carb, moderate protein smoothie.

Makes: 2 servings
Serving size: 4 oz.

**Nutritional Information** (Per serving):

Calories: 252
Fat: 18 g
Carbohydrates: 5 g
Protein: 17 g

**All you need:**

½ cup unsweetened almond milk, vanilla
½ cup half and half
½ avocado, peeled, pitted, sliced
1 tbsp. almond butter
1 scoop Isopure Zero Carb protein powder
Pinch of cinnamon
½ tsp vanilla extract
2-4 ice cubes
Liquid stevia, to sweeten

**All you do:**

Add all ingredients into blender and blend until smooth.

# STRAWBERRY ALMOND DELIGHT

A high fat, low carb, moderate protein smoothie.

Makes: 2 servings
Serving size: 10 oz.

**Nutritional Information** (Per serving):

Calories: 304
Fat: 25 g
Carbohydrates: 7 g
Protein: 15 g

**All you need:**

16 oz. unsweetened almond milk, vanilla
1 packet stevia
4 oz. heavy cream
1 scoop Whey Isolate Vanilla protein powder
¼ cup frozen strawberries, unsweetened

**All you do:**

Add all ingredients into blender and blend until smooth.

# CREAMY BLACKBERRY

A high fat, low carb, low protein shake. Ensure to meet your daily protein meal requirements per meal through other dietary sources.

Makes: 2 servings
Serving size: 4 oz.

**Nutritional Information** (Per serving):

Calories: 237.5
Fat: 22 g
Carbohydrates: 6 g
Protein: 2.3 g

## All you need:

1 cup fresh blackberries
1 cup ice cubes
Liquid stevia, to sweeten
¾ cup heavy whipping cream

## All you do:

Add all ingredients into blender and blend until smooth.

# PEANUT BUTTER MILKSHAKE

A high fat, moderate carbs, low protein shake. Ensure to meet your daily protein meal requirements through other dietary sources.

Makes: 2 servings
Serving size: approximately 1 cup

**Nutritional Information** (Per serving):

Calories: 253
Fat: 23.8 g
Carbohydrates: 7 g
Protein: 5.5 g

**All you need:**

½ cup coconut milk, regular
1 cup unsweetened almond milk, vanilla
2 tbsp. all natural peanut butter
1 tsp vanilla extract
1 cup ice cubes
1 packet stevia

**All you do:**

Add all ingredients into blender and blend until smooth.

# RASPBERRY SMOOTHIE

A high fat, moderate carbs, moderate to high protein smoothie, depending on your daily protein meal requirements.

Makes: 2 serving
Serving size: 4-5 oz.

**Nutritional Information** (Per serving):

Calories: 285
Fat: 22 g
Carbohydrates: 7 g
Protein: 14.5 g

**All you need:**

½ cup fresh raspberries
1 cup unsweetened almond milk, vanilla
1 scoop prebiotic fibre (Pinnaclife Prebiotic Fibre)
1 scoop Vanilla Whey Isolate protein powder
2 tbsp. coconut oil
¼ cup coconut flakes, unsweetened
3-4 ice cubes

**All you do:**

Add all ingredients into blender and blend until smooth.

# LEPRECHAUN SHAKE

An all-around moderate fat, carb and low to moderate protein shake.

Makes: 2 servings
Serving size: 5 oz.

**Nutritional Information** (Per serving):

Calories: 217
Fat: 13 g
Carbohydrates: 7.5 g
Protein: 13 g

**All you need:**

½ avocado, peeled, pitted, sliced
¼ cup unsweetened coconut milk
Small bunch of baby spinach
¼ cup fresh mint
1 scoop Isopure Zero Carb Whey Protein Isolate
1 tsp vanilla extract
Liquid stevia, to sweeten
Water, if desired
2-3 ice cubes, if desired

**All you do:**

Halve and peel avocado. Add avocado and remaining ingredients into blender and blend until smooth.

# BREAKFAST EGG SMOOTHIE

A moderate carb, high fat, higher protein smoothie, for those with higher protein requirements.

Makes: 2 servings
Serving size: 4-5 oz.

**Nutritional Information** (Per serving):

Calories: 266
Fat: 17 g
Carbohydrates: 6.3 g
Protein: 22.6 g

**All you need:**

½ cup coconut milk, unsweetened
½ cup Lifeway Organic Whole Milk Kefir, plain
4 tbsp. chia seeds
1 oz. egg substitute dry powder

**All you do:**

Add all ingredients into blender and blend until smooth.

# PEANUT BUTTER CARAMEL SHAKE

A high fat, moderate carbs, low protein shake. Ensure to meet your daily protein meal requirements through other dietary sources.

Makes: 1 serving
Serving size: 8 oz.

**Nutritional Information** (Per serving):

Calories: 366
Fat: 35 g
Carbohydrates: 6 g
Protein: 7 g

**All you need:**

1 cup ice cubes
1 cup coconut milk, unsweetened
2 tbsp. natural peanut butter
2 tbsp. Sugar-free Torani Salted Caramel
¼ tsp. xanthan gum, to thicken smoothie
1 tbsp. MCT oil

**All you do:**

Add all ingredients into blender and blend until smooth.

Skye Howard

# SMOOTHIES & SHAKES
# 8G - 10G CARBS

### CREAMY GREEN MACHINE 38
Calories: 279
Fat: 18 g
Carbohydrates: 9 g
Protein: 18 g

### COCONUT SUPERFOOD SMOOTHIE 39
Calories: 272
Fat: 22 g
Carbohydrates: 8 g
Protein: 15 g

### CREAMY STRAWBERRY 40
Calories:  133.5
Fat: 39 g
Carbohydrates: 9.5 g
Protein: 27 g

### SPRING SMOOTHIE 41
Calories: 263
Fat: 19 g
Carbohydrates: 10 g
Protein: 12 g

## VANILLA HEMP 42
Calories: 250
Fat: 20.5 g
Carbohydrates: 9.5 g
Protein: 7 g

## CACAO SUPER SMOOTHIE 43
Calories: 445
Fat: 14 g
Carbohydrates: 9 g
Protein: 16 g

## PEPPERMINT MOCHA 44
Calories: 198
Fat: 16 g
Carbohydrates: 9 g
Protein: 3 g

## HAPPY GUT SMOOTHIE 45
Calories: 409
Fat: 33 g
Carbohydrates: 8 g
Protein: 12 g

## STRAWBERRY CHEESECAKE SMOOTHIE 46
Calories: 247
Fat: 19 g
Carbohydrates: 8 g
Protein: 3 g

## SILKEN TOFU SMOOTHIE                    47
Calories: 208
Fat: 12 g
Carbohydrates: 10 g
Protein: 18 g


## BLUEBERRY BANANA BREAD                 48
Calories: 507
Fat: 48 g
Carbohydrates: 10 g
Protein: 9 g


## MANGO GREEN TEA & CARROT SMOOTHIE    49
Calories: 133
Fat: 9 g
Carbohydrates: 10 g
Protein: 6 g


## PUMPKIN PARADISE                       50
Calories: 268
Fat: 10.5 g
Carbohydrates: 9.5 g
Protein: 29 g


## CREAMY GREEN SMOOTHIE                  51
Calories: 316
Fat: 25.8 g
Carbohydrates: 10.5 g
Protein: 13 g

# CREAMY GREEN MACHINE

A high fat, moderate carb (depending on your daily carb limit), moderate to higher protein smoothie, for those with higher Protein requirements.

Makes: 2 servings
Serving size: 8 oz.

**Nutritional Information** (Per serving):

Calories: 279
Fat: 18 g
Carbohydrates: 9 g
Protein: 18 g

**All you need:**

½ cup unsweetened almond milk, vanilla
½ cup half and half
½ avocado, peeled, pitted, sliced
½ cup frozen blueberries, unsweetened
1 cup spinach
1 tbsp. almond butter
1 scoop Isopure Zero Carb protein powder
2-4 ice cubes
1 packet stevia

**All you do:**

Add all ingredients into blender and blend until smooth.

# COCONUT SUPERFOOD SMOOTHIE

A high fat, moderate carb (depending on your daily carb limit), moderate protein smoothie, for those with higher protein requirements.

Makes: 2 servings
Serving size: 6 oz.

**Nutritional Information** (Per serving):

Calories: 272
Fat: 22 g
Carbohydrates: 8 g
Protein: 15 g

**All you need:**

½ cup unsweetened almond milk, vanilla
½ cup coconut cream
1 scoop Isopure Zero Carb protein powder
½ cup frozen blueberries, unsweetened
2-4 ice cubes

**All you do:**

Add all ingredients into blender and blend until smooth.

For added protein, add in 1 scoop of Isopure Zero Carb protein powder for 25 g.

# CREAMY STRAWBERRY

A high fat, moderate carb (depending on your daily carb limit), higher protein smoothie, for those with higher protein requirements.

Makes: 2 servings
Serving size: 1 cup

**Nutritional Information** (Per serving):

Calories:  133.5
Fat: 39 g
Carbohydrates: 9.5 g
Protein: 27 g

**All you need:**

1 cup ice cubes
½ cup water
1 scoop Isopure Zero Carb Strawberry protein powder
3 slices avocado, peeled, pitted
1 oz. MCT oil
1/2 cup frozen strawberries, unsweetened

**All you do:**

Add all ingredients into blender and blend until smooth.

# SPRING SMOOTHIE

A high fat, moderate carb (depending on your daily carb limit), lower protein smoothie.

Makes: 2 servings
Serving size: 8 oz.

**Nutritional Information** (Per serving):
Calories: 263
Fat: 19 g
Carbohydrates: 10 g
Protein: 12 g

**All you need:**

2 large handfuls mixed greens (spinach and kale)
1 oz. almonds, unsalted
¼ cup frozen blueberries, unsweetened
1 tbsp. chia seeds
1 cup raspberry tea, unsweetened

**All you do:**

Add all ingredients into blender and blend until smooth.

# VANILLA HEMP

A high fat, moderate carb (depending on your daily carb limit), low protein smoothie. Ensure to meet your daily protein meal requirements through other dietary sources.

Makes: 2 serving
Serving size: 8 oz.

**Nutritional Information** (Per serving):

Calories: 250
Fat: 20.5 g
Carbohydrates: 9.5 g
Protein: 7 g

**All you need:**

1 cup water
1 cup unsweetened hemp milk, vanilla
1 ½ tbsp. coconut oil, unrefined
½ cup frozen berries, mixed
4 cup leafy greens (kale and spinach)
1 tbsp. flaxseeds or chia seeds
1 tbsp. almond butter

**All you do:**

Add all ingredients into blender and blend until smooth.

# CACAO SUPER SMOOTHIE

A high fat, moderate carb (depending on your daily carb limit), moderate protein smoothie, depending on your daily protein requirements.

Makes: 2 servings
Serving size: 10 oz.

**Nutritional Information** (Per serving):

Calories: 445
Fat: 14 g
Carbohydrates: 9 g
Protein: 16 g

**All you need:**

½ cup unsweetened almond milk, vanilla
½ cup half and half
½ avocado, peeled, pitted, sliced
½ cup frozen blueberries, unsweetened
1 tbsp. cacao powder
1 scoop Whey Isolate Vanilla protein powder
Liquid stevia, to sweeten

**All you do:**

Add all ingredients into blender and blend until smooth.

# PEPPERMINT MOCHA

A moderate fat, moderate carb (depending on your daily carb limit) and very low protein smoothie. Ensure to meet your daily protein meal intake through other dietary sources.

Makes: 2 servings
Serving size: 6 oz.

**Nutritional Information** (Per serving):

Calories: 198
Fat: 16 g
Carbohydrates: 9 g
Protein: 3 g

**All you need:**

1 cup cold coffee
1/3 Organic Chocolove Dark Chocolate, 73%
2 tbsp. avocado, peeled, pitted, sliced
½ cup half and half
2 tbsp. fresh mint (about 20 leaves) or 1 tsp mint extract
2 tsp cacao powder
¼ cup water
Liquid stevia, to sweetener
¼ cup ice cubes

**All you do:**

In a medium saucepan, heat chocolate over low heat then stir in half and half, water, cacao and liquid stevia.

Add remaining ingredients into blender with chocolate mixture and blend until smooth.

# HAPPY GUT SMOOTHIE

A high fat, lower carb (depending on your daily carb limit) low protein smoothie. Ensure to meet your daily meal protein intake through other dietary sources.

Makes: 1 serving
Serving size: 10 oz.

**Nutritional Information** (Per serving):

Calories: 409
Fat: 33 g
Carbohydrates: 8 g
Protein: 12 g

**All you need:**

2-3 cup spinach leaves
1 ½ tbsp. coconut oil, unrefined
½ cup plain full fat yogurt
1 tbsp. chia seeds
1 serving aloe vera leaves
½ cup frozen blueberries, unsweetened
1 tbsp. hemp hearts
1 cup water
1 scoop Pinnaclife Prebiotic Fibre

**All you do:**

Add all ingredients into blender and blend until smooth.

# STRAWBERRY CHEESECAKE SMOOTHIE

A high fat, lower carb (depending upon your daily carb limit) and very low protein (3g) smoothie. Ensure to meet your daily protein meal intake through other dietary sources.

Makes: 1 serving
Serving size: 4 oz.

**Nutritional Information** (Per serving):

Calories: 247
Fat: 19 g
Carbohydrates: 8 g
Protein: 3 g

**All you need:**

½ cup frozen strawberries, unsweetened
½ cup unsweetened vanilla almond milk
Liquid stevia, to sweeten
½ tsp vanilla extract
2 oz. cream cheese, regular
3-4 ice cubes
Water, optional

**All you do:**

Add all ingredients into blender and blend until smooth.

Add 1 scoop of Isopure Zero Carb protein powder for higher protein intake, if desired.

# SILKEN TOFU SMOOTHIE

A lower fat, moderate carb (depending on your daily carb limit) and moderate protein smoothie.

Makes: 2 servings
Serving size: 5 oz.

**Nutritional Information** (Per serving):

Calories: 208
Fat: 12 g
Carbohydrates: 10 g
Protein: 18 g

**All you need:**

½ cup strawberries, unfrozen
Silken tofu
1 cup unsweetened almond milk, vanilla
Pinch of cinnamon
Liquid Stevia, to sweeten

**All you do:**

Add all ingredients into blender and blend until smooth.

# BLUEBERRY BANANA BREAD

A high fat, moderate carb (depending on your daily carb limit), and low protein smoothie. Ensure to meet your daily meal protein requirement through other dietary sources.

Makes: 2 servings
Serving size: 5 oz.

**Nutritional Information** (Per serving):

Calories: 507
Fat: 48 g
Carbohydrates: 10 g
Protein: 9 g

**All you need:**

3 tbsp. ground flaxseed
1 tbsp. chia seeds, whole
1 cup coconut milk
Liquid stevia, to sweeten
¼ cup frozen blueberries, unsweetened
1 tbsp. MCT oil
1 ½ tsp banana extract, McCormick's
2 tbsp. almond meal

**All you do:**

Add all ingredients into blender and blend until smooth.

# MANGO GREEN TEA & CARROT SMOOTHIE

A lower fat, moderate carb (depending on your daily carb limit), low protein smoothie. Ensure to meet your daily meal protein intake through other dietary sources.

Makes: 2 servings
Serving size: 8 oz.

**Nutritional Information** (Per serving):

Calories: 133
Fat: 9 g
Carbohydrates: 10 g
Protein: 6 g

**All you need:**

2 cup water
½ cup baby carrots
Pinch of fresh ginger
½ cup frozen mango
Liquid stevia, to sweeten
1 tbsp. chia seed

**All you do:**

Add all ingredients into blender and blend until smooth.

# PUMPKIN PARADISE

A lower fat, moderate carb (depending on your daily carb limit), higher protein smoothie, for those with higher protein requirements. To increase the fat add 1 tbsp. (15ml) MCT Oil. 1 tbsp. contains 100 calories, provides 100 calories from fat, with a total fat content of 14g (saturated).

Makes: 1 serving
Serving size: 6 oz.

**Nutritional Information** (Per serving):

Calories: 268
Fat: 10.5 g
Carbohydrates: 9.5 g
Protein: 29 g

**All you need:**

½ cup unsweetened almond milk, vanilla
½ cup water
½ cup canned pumpkin
½ tsp pumpkin pie spice
Stevia packet
1 scoop Isopure Zero Carb protein powder
1 oz. cream cheese
2-3 ice cubes
Ground cinnamon, to taste

**All you do:**

Add all ingredients into blender and blend until smooth. Top with a sprinkle of cinnamon, if desired.

# CREAMY GREEN SMOOTHIE

A high fat, moderate carb (depending on your daily carb limit), low to moderate protein smoothie.

Makes: 2 serving
Serving size: approximately 1 cup

**Nutritional Information** (Per serving):

Calories: 316
Fat: 25.8 g
Carbohydrates: 10.5 g
Protein: 13 g

**All you need:**

¼ avocado, peeled, pitted, sliced
4 broccoli florets, if desired
1 bunch of kale and spinach
1 slice honeydew
½ cup coconut milk
2 tbsp. plain Greek yogurt, full fat
1 tbsp. almond butter
½ cup unsweetened almond milk, vanilla
¼ cup water, optional
½ scoop Isopure Zero Carb Protein powder

**All you do:**

Blend vegetables and nuts first then add in remaining ingredients; blend until smooth. For added crunch, garnish the top with a few a walnuts, if desired.

Skye Howard

.

# SMOOTHIES & SHAKES
# 11G - 15G CARBS

## FOR THOSE WITH HIGHER DAILY CARB LIMITS

BANANA ALMOND SMOOTHIE                    55
Calories: 89
Fat: 5 g
Carbohydrates: 11.5 g
Protein: 2.2 g


KICKING KALE SHAKE                        56
Calories: 164.5
Fat: 11 g
Carbohydrates: 10.7g
Protein: 3 g


RED VELVET SMOOTHIE                       57
Calories: 228
Fat: 16 g
Carbohydrates: 13 g
Protein: 7 g


ENDURANCE BEET SMOOTHIE                   58
Calories: 396
Fat: 26 g
Carbohydrates: 15 g
Protein: 26 g


WHIPPED SHAKE                             59
Calories: 238
Fat: 22 g
Carbohydrates: 13 g
Protein: 6.3 g

## CHOCOLATE CHIP BANANA SMOOTHIE          60

Calories: 307.5
Fat: 26.5 g
Carbohydrates: 13 g
Protein: 7.2 g

# BANANA ALMOND SMOOTHIE

A low fat, moderate carb (depending on your daily carb limit), very low protein smoothie. Ensure to meet your daily meal protein requirements through other dietary sources. For increased fat add one tbsp. (15ml) MCT oil. 1 tbsp. contains 100 calories, provides 100 calories from fat, with a total fat content of 14g (saturated).

Makes: 2 servings
Serving size: 4 oz.

**Nutritional Information** (Per serving):

Calories: 89
Fat: 5 g
Carbohydrates: 11.5 g
Protein: 2.2 g

**All you need:**

1 banana, under ripe, small, frozen (under ripe bananas are abundant in prebiotic fiber)
1 cup spinach
¾ cup unsweetened almond milk, vanilla
1 tbsp. almond butter

**All you do:**

Add all ingredients into blender and blend until smooth.

# KICKING KALE SHAKE

A lower fat, moderate carb (depending upon your daily carb limit), very low protein shake. Ensure to meet your daily protein meal intake through other dietary sources. To increase fat add one tbsp. (15ml) MCT oil. 1 tbsp. contains 100 calories, provides 100 calories from fat, with a total fat content of 14g (saturated).

Makes: 1 serving
Serving size: 8 oz.

**Nutritional Information** (Per serving, without protein powder):

Calories: 164.5
Fat: 11 g
Carbohydrates: 10.7g
Protein: 3 g

**All you need:**

1 small sweet potato, cooked, cooled, sliced
¾ cup unsweetened almond milk, vanilla
½ tsp ground cinnamon
¼ tsp ground allspice
¼ tsp ground nutmeg
1 tsp pure vanilla extract
2 slices avocado, peeled, pitted, sliced
Liquid stevia, to taste
1 scoop Isopure Zero Carb protein powder, if desired

**All you do:**

Add all ingredients into blender and blend until smooth.

# RED VELVET SMOOTHIE

A moderate fat, moderate carb (depending upon your daily carb limit), low protein smoothie. Ensure to meet your daily protein meal requirement through other dietary sources.

Makes: 2 servings
Serving size: 9 oz.

**Nutritional Information** (Per serving):

Calories: 228
Fat: 16 g
Carbohydrates: 13 g
Protein: 7 g

**All you need:**

2 cup unsweetened almond milk, vanilla
2 cup ice cubes
2-3 slices avocado, peeled, pitted, sliced
1 beet, small, cooked
2 tbsp. cacao
¼ tsp pure vanilla extract
Liquid stevia, to sweeten

**All you do:**

Add all ingredients into blender and blend until smooth.

# ENDURANCE BEET SMOOTHIE

A high fat, moderate to high carb (depending on your daily carb limit), higher protein smoothie.

Makes: 1 serving
Serving size: 16 oz.

**Nutritional Information** (Per serving, with MCT Oil):

Calories: 396
Fat: 26 g
Carbohydrates: 15 g
Protein: 26 g

**All you need:**

1 small beet, cooked
1 oz. walnuts
Pinch of cinnamon
Small piece fresh ginger
1 scoop Unjury Unflavored Protein
1 cup unsweetened almond milk
1 cup cold water
1 small carrot, sliced
2 slices red apple
1 tbsp. MCT oil, optional

**All you do:**

Add all ingredients into blender and blend until smooth.

# WHIPPED SHAKE

A high fat, low to moderate carb (depending upon your daily carb limit), low protein shake. Ensure to meet your daily meal protein intake through other dietary sources.

Makes: 1 serving
Serving size: 10 oz.

**Nutritional Information** (Per serving):

Calories: 238
Fat: 22 g
Carbohydrates: 13 g
Protein: 6.3 g

**All you need:**

1 cup unsweetened almond milk
1/3 cup heavy whipping cream
2-4 drops liquid stevia
½ tsp vanilla extract
2 tbsp. cacao (use 1 tbsp. for lower carbohydrate)
3 ice cubes

**All you do:**

Add all ingredients into blender and blend until smooth.

# CHOCOLATE CHIP BANANA SMOOTHIE

A high fat, moderate to high carb (depending upon your daily carb limit), moderate protein smoothie.

Makes: 6 servings
Serving size: 4-5 oz.

**Nutritional Information** (Per serving):

Calories: 307.5
Fat: 26.5 g
Carbohydrates: 13 g
Protein: 7.2 g

**All you need:**

1 frozen medium banana, under ripe, sliced (under ripe bananas are abundant in prebiotic fibre)
1 cup almond butter
Liquid stevia, to taste
2 tbsp. cacao powder
½ cup Enjoy Life Dairy-Free Chocolate Chips
2 cups unsweetened almond milk, vanilla
2 cup ice cubes

**All you do:**

Add all ingredients into blender and blend until smooth.

# ALSO BY SKYE HOWARD FOR THE KETOGENIC DIET:

## Keto Make Ahead Freezer Meals & Snacks

## Keto One Pot Meals

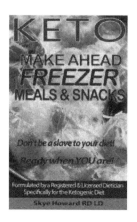 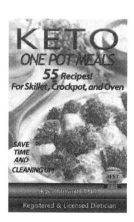

# ALSO BY SCG PUBLISHING

Chilli Jam Recipes by Amanda Kent

The Migraine Diet Cookbook by Michelle Strong

Migraine Diet Smoothies by Michelle Strong

HIIT: High Intensity Interval Training - Look Like an Athlete, Feel Like an Athlete by Steve Ryan

29587374R00042

Made in the USA
Middletown, DE
27 December 2018